Back Pain Relief –
While You Sleep

How your sleep position can fix your neck, shoulders and back

James Hughes

Copyright © 2017 James Hughes

All rights reserved.

ISBN: 1977628680
ISBN-13: 9781977628688

CONTENTS

1 INTRODUCTION

This is the story of how I beat my bad back – by changing what I did at night.

Doctors think I inherited my bad back (thanks Dad…). Some days it has been so bad that my legs go numb and I just can't find a position that is comfortable.

But I know that I'm lucky. Some people have it far worse – and if you are one of them then you have my sincere sympathies.

I hope that this is book is one step on your way to finding some long-term relief from one of the most widespread, horrible and debilitating conditions that there is.

Nine out of ten adults will experience it at some point in their lives.

I tried everything to solve my backpain: one of those special chairs that it's far too easy to fall off (and which make your knees ache), medication – I even considered surgery just to get some relief.

When it was at its worst, I had just become a dad for the first time and, throughout the long, drawn out process I kept thinking that, when our daughter was a toddler, I wouldn't be able to lift her up because my pain would be too great.

It was one of the most depressing images I kept returning to in my mind: me badly wanting to scoop her up, out of danger and into my arms but not being able to. What sort of dad would that make me?

So I was pretty desperate to try anything and everything.

One of the things I tried was a pilates evening class. This isn't a book about that but, as an aside, if you haven't tried pilates yet then it's worth signing up to your local group and giving it a go.

It really helped me. And it's where this breakthrough came from.

One evening, as I lay on the floor, stretching, it occurred to me... what I was doing wasn't a hundred miles away from the position I sleep in.

So I thought: rather than lying here for twenty minutes a day or perhaps once a week at an exercise class, wouldn't it make more sense to do the stretch for eight hours a night?

(OK, I admit, some of this was me being lazy and thinking that I could get the stretches out the way while I was fast asleep and do something more interesting with my waking hours instead).

Because I had been sent to see so many specialists, doctors, physiotherapists and chiropractors I mentioned the idea to a couple of them.

And both said the same thing: too many people sleep in the wrong position.

They told me, if people slept in the right way during the night they would find they had far fewer aches and pains during the day.

So I did some more research, had some more conversations – and then tried it out.

Do you know what? They're right.

It *is* possible to alleviate your back pain by changing the position you sleep in. You just need to know what is right for your condition.

So, if you have back, neck or shoulder pain then this book is for you.

It sets out, simply and clearly, what you need to do to get a good night's sleep – and a day which isn't blighted by pain.

This book will tell you not only what position to switch to in order to take the strain off your body, but also how to check whether your mattress and pillow is helping or hindering your recovery.

It tells you the worst possible position for you to sleep in, wherever your pain is centered. It tells you why pillows don't always need to go under your head (and the one sleeping position where they should *never* go under your head).

Plus, the one thing that most of us do in bed which increases the strain on our neck by six times.

The position that we start the night off in, of course, isn't necessarily the same that we end the night in. We all toss and turn, moving about the bed and shifting position.

In fact, sleep studies by researchers have found that, on average, we each change position twelve times a night (although that number declines as we grow older).

But the fact remains that, if you are able to make a change to how you start off the night, it is very likely to have an impact on your health and wellbeing.

I wanted to write a book that everyone is able to read, immediately understand and use this very evening to help you move forward on your road to recovery.

I hope it helps you.

Oh, and now our daughter is a toddler, turns out that I definitely can pick her up for a cuddle.

Good luck – and good sleeping!

2 SHOULDER PAIN

Humans are creatures of habit. We all have things we do every night, often in the same order. We brush our teeth, we undress and, crucially, we often choose to sleep on the same side.

If that sounds like you, it could be doing your body more harm than good.

Not the toothbrushing (your dentist will be pleased to hear it) but automatically turning onto the same side night after night after night.

Think about how long we spend in bed. Let's say you get the mythical eight hours that experts are always telling us is so important.

That means that, over the course of a year, you are spending the equivalent of more than 120 days with your body weight resting on the same side.

Now, in reality, with the tossing and turning that we all do every night, it will be much less than that. But having a "default" position could still be storing up some big problems.

Before we come onto what you can do about the pain if you are already suffering from it, let's pause to work out what is going on inside you.

You will have a sense – however hazy – of what your shoulder joint looks like. There is a ball and socket joint, surrounded by a load of muscles and tendons which are used to stabilize the joint. It is known as the "cuff."

These muscles and tendons can be damaged if you suffer an accident such as a fall. But they can also take a pounding from repeated stress – such as being repeatedly slept on.

Internally, night after night, tendons are being pressed against the underlying bone. This causes inflammation and is known as rotator cuff tendinitis or impingement syndrome.

You may have noticed some stiffness in the shoulder at first – even some mild pain. This is especially noticeable when you put pressure on your shoulder or lift your arm.

You can tell if you have rotator cuff tendinitis because the pain is usually located at the front of the shoulder but then stops again just before the elbow.

Sound familiar?

That's the science bit. Now here is what you can do to stop it.

The good news is that it is relatively easy. If it started because you were sleeping on one side more than the other then it can be fixed by doing the opposite.

Try changing your position to the other side. Over time that should take the pressure off your body and allow it to heal itself.

You are probably ahead of me on the drawback to this. Over time you are going to end up sleeping on the other side... and the whole sorry situation will start up again.

So, here is the more difficult, long-term solution: Change the way you sleep completely.

If you really can't because you are a side sleeper through and through then make sure that you keep switching sides.

Another tip is to move your pillow higher up, which should mean that there is less pressure on your shoulder (there is much more to come on picking the right pillow for you in a later chapter, by the way).

Pull your legs up slightly towards your chest and pop another pillow between your knees. This means that you are also keeping your spine and pelvis in the best alignment.

Give it a try and see how you get on. It will feel weird. But it will feel a lot better than the pain that you are currently enduring.

Otherwise you might want to try keeping the joint as immobile as possible during the day and treating it with an icepack to try to take down the inflammation.

Of course, if your shoulder is still playing up after a few weeks of trying to fix it yourself then it is worth making an appointment with your doctor to make sure that there is not anything else going on in the background.

In an ideal world you would change your sleeping position to your back.

I know that is easier said than done – as a side sleeper myself the thought of changing that now is difficult.

There are some things that you can do to make it easier and to ensure that you are in the right position.

First, find a thin or orthopedic pillow and put it under your head as you lie on your back.

Then take a second pillow and hug it to your stomach. That should ensure that your shoulders are kept in the correct position.

Whatever you do, don't switch to sleeping on your front because that has the potential to end up with misalignment of your shoulders (among many other negatives).

While you wait for your change in sleep position to have the desired effect, check what sort of pain medication you are using.

Because the pain is coming from inflammation you want to make sure you are using an anti-inflammatory painkiller. Anything that isn't anti-inflammatory isn't going to be doing the job for you.

Finally, if you are in a lot of pain, switch to a reclining chair for a few nights while you wait for things to settle down.

Check in with your doctor because, in severe cases, you can have injections or have a conversation about surgery.

3 BACK PAIN

Back pain is one of those conditions that you feel almost completely alone in, but that couldn't be further from the truth.

More than 80% of adults will suffer back pain at some point in their lives. And, when it hits, does it knock you for six!

The nightmare is that, as well as being with you during the day, it is also there, in the background, at night.

And that is where it starts getting really tricky.

When you aren't getting a good night's sleep it makes the next day even harder work – even before you factor in the pain.

And then you are worrying about getting to sleep in the evening. Which makes it harder to drop off. And then the whole cycle feels like it is going on.

And on.

And on.

So, here is how to break the vicious circle and get back to having a good night's sleep… and reduce the pain.

The most important thing you need to do is maintain the normal curvature of your spine.

Having a very soft mattress will not be helping with that. So ask yourself some tough questions about how long you have had your mattress and whether it still suits your needs.

If it is between seven and ten years old then it is probably time to replace it. Ditto if you can hear it creaking or groaning when you are trying to get some rest.

When I first moved in with my girlfriend (now my wife) it took me a few months to discover that her ultra-soft mattress was, in fact, second hand from the local market.

We changed it, bought a new one and, within a few nights, my back pain had improved significantly. It was being made worse by the softness of the mattress.

Now, there is a big myth that if you have back pain what you really want is a hard mattress. The harder the better. In fact, why not sleep on the floor and cut out the mattress altogether?

You hear stories about people sleeping on piles of bricks – or even taking a door off its hinges and using that.

I'm not sure where this has come from because, if you think about it, the same rules apply to hard mattresses as apply to their too-soft counterparts.

You want a mattress that is going to maintain the normal curvature of your spine. A mattress that is too hard isn't going to do that for you… even if you feel that it *must* be doing you good because it is so uncomfortable.

In reality all that you are doing is creating pressure points – a surefire way of producing extra aches and pains on top of the ones that you have already got.

So, ignore anyone (especially bed salespeople!) who tell you that what you need is a hard mattress. Look instead for one that keeps your head, shoulders, hips and feet in proper alignment.

And above all – test it out.

When I say test it out, I don't just mean get up onto the bed in the showroom and roll around on it for a couple of minutes.

I mean test it out, properly, in your own home. By (would you believe it?) actually sleeping on it.

Remember my experience when I moved in with my girlfriend? It took me a few nights – probably weeks – to know for sure that the new mattress had solved the problem.

Most reputable mattress makes/bed sellers now offer a decent trial period during which you can send the mattress back. A hundred nights seems to be a fairly popular duration.

Look out for these trials and make full use of them. But, a word of warning, some companies have pretty steep costs to make a return. So do your homework first.

Once you have got your mattress sorted, it is also worth looking at your pillow because a lot of the same rules apply.

For more on this check out the chapter on neck pain because (surprise, surprise) it's generally the neck that will bear the brunt of an imperfect pillow.

But, before we leave your bedroom set-up, it is worth considering how you get out bed.

I know. But bear with me.

Most people get out of bed by sitting up and then, crucially, twisting their back in order to put their feet on the floor – and then using their back to push themselves up.

You may not ever have thought about this before – especially if you aren't a morning person. But it is worth paying attention to how much strain you put on your back first thing.

So, tomorrow, try this: roll onto your side at the edge of your bed from whatever position you are sleeping in. Use your arm to push yourself up and swing your legs over, ensuring that you use them to push yourself up, rather than your back.

Onto the all-important question of how to sleep to minimize your back pain.

And it isn't what you would expect.

If you have got pain in your back then the sensible thing to do is to avoid lying on your back, right?

Wrong.

Assuming that you have a decent mattress that keeps your spine in alignment, you could do a lot worse than trying to sleep on your back as often as possible.

That way you are spending up to eight hours a day with your back in near perfect alignment.

To help with that, place a pillow under your knees to help restore the natural curve of the spine and reduce tension in your tendons.

Add a small, rolled-up towel under your lower back too.

Yes, it may take some getting used to.

So, why does sleeping on your back make sense when you actually have back problems?

It is because your weight is being evenly distributed across the widest area of your body. That means that you have less chance of putting strain on pressure points.

If you just can't get used to sleeping on your back then there are some more options to consider.

For stomach sleepers it is worth placing a pillow under your abdomen and pelvis so that the small of your back does not move forward.

Some people may find they do not need a pillow under their head in this position.

This position may be especially useful for those suffering degenerative disc disease since it relieves stress being put on the space between your discs.

But stomach sleeping comes with a health warning. Not only does it flatten the natural curvature of your spine but it also artificially rotates your neck.

There is much more on neck pain to come – but it is worth noting here that sleeping on your front could make this worse or result in back pain between your shoulder blades.

For side sleepers, pull your knees up a little towards your chest. Place a small pillow between your knees. This should help take some of the load off your lower back.

A word of warning. Don't always pick the same side. The more that you end up resting on one particular shoulder or the other, the greater the chances that you will develop further aches and pains.

Don't neglect adding the pillow between your knees. Even though it sounds like more trouble than it is worth, it is actually the pillow that is doing the trick in this position.

It is keeping your hips, pelvis and spine in better alignment. And that, after all, is what we are trying to achieve.

If you have a herniated disc then pull your knees up even tighter to your chest and go for the full fetal position.

Because your discs are effectively cushioning the vertebrae in your spine, one being pushed out of alignment can lead to anything from weakness to nerve pain.

Curling your torso towards your knees in the fetal position allows you to reopen the space between the vertebrae.

One word here on reclining chairs. Some with back pain find that these are the comfiest way of getting some rest.

Although a recliner is not necessarily the best choice in the long-term, it can help if you suffer from isthmic spondylolisthesis.

This is a condition whereby one vertebrae slips over those below. As you lean backwards it creates an angle that helps reduce the pressure on your spine.

It is why some bed makers now manufacture adjustable mattresses that allow you to find the most comfortable position for you.

Whatever your back condition and whichever sleeping position you choose, the key always is to ensure that you keep your body in alignment.

To check on your alignment focus on your ears, shoulders and hips.

Gaps between your body and bed should be filled in with pillows in order to reduce the stress.

Finally, consider how you change position in bed. Clearly you can't do anything when you are asleep. But as you toss and turn trying to get comfortable, try not to put extra strain on your body.

It is all too easy to accidentally twist yourself out of alignment. Try to make sure that you turn your whole body together.

Pull your knees up to your chest a little as you roll over.

4 NECK PAIN

Just as we started the last chapter by checking whether you are sleeping on the right mattress, this one begins by making sure your pillow isn't causing more problems than it's worth.

Most people are willing to spend some time (and money!) on getting the right mattress. It's going to look after your back, right? But fewer invest in making sure they have the right pillow.

In fact, even fewer know what the right pillow is and how to use it.

Standby – you're about to join a very select group.

How do you know if it's time for a new pillow? Well, if you're getting neck pain you could do worse than to think about a replacement.

But here's a clever test that could help make up your mind. If you have a traditional fiberfill pillow try folding it in half and putting a heavy book on top of it.

If it springs back into shape then you're all good. But if it stays folded in half it might be time to go shopping.

Similarly, memory foam pillows that are going crumbly (and don't we all over time…?) or that struggle to hold their shape are going to be on their way out.

If you are worried about allergens then you probably want to replace your pillow every eighteen months in any case.

Yep, eighteen months. Your pillow harbors all sorts of nasties. I'm not going to scare you too much by listing them all.

But I will just mention dust mites and mold…

So, now you have decided to replace your pillow, what is the right sort for you?

Firstly, and most importantly, you are looking for a pillow that fits with the way you sleep.

Make sure that, whatever position you are in, your pillow cradles your head and neck. If it isn't, then it isn't supporting the upper portion of your spine.

Ideally you want to ensure that your neck aligns with your spine (that word – alignment – again!) in a neutral position while you drop off to sleep.

And if you are used to having the pillow under your shoulders – do yourself a favor and stop right now!

If you sleep on your back then you want a pillow that completely fills the space between your mattress and your neck.

You might also want to try using a couple of thinner pillows rather than one big fluffy one. Alternatively, look out for more specialist offerings.

One possibility is a pillow that has stuffed extra padding into the bottom to provide extra support for the neck. Or look at memory foam (although not necessarily one of the brand names).

This material effectively moulds itself to your neck, although they can feel bigger and thicker. A water pillow could be an option to give good overall support.

Sleep on your stomach? Hmm... can I persuade you to try another position? As we've discovered, it probably isn't doing you any good in the long-term.

If I can't, then look for the thinnest pillow possible. Or even no pillow at all.

Or, if you want to break out of the habit of stomach sleeping, look for a body pillow. That way you can sleep on your side while holding the pillow, giving you the impression of something against your stomach.

That could be enough to move you into a healthier sleeping position. Got to be worth a go, right?

Side sleepers will want to find a thicker, firmer pillow – especially one that minimizes the gap between your ear and shoulder.

Couple that with another firm pillow, but this one between your knees. You can use a rolled up towel instead if you would prefer.

Other types of pillows it might be worth investigating are hybrid pillows. These have a memory foam core but are surrounded with a softer layer.

You end up with both support and comfort and, even better, the pillow can adapt as you switch positions during your sleep.

Oh – and I mentioned memory foam earlier? Some sleep experts now do not recommend the first generation ones. You will recognize the unconventional shape and double hump. One expert described it as "too one dimensional."

Just as you test out a new mattress, try to test out your new pillow.

Manufacturers don't tend to give you a free trial in the same way as they do a new mattress, but you might be able to give it a go in the store.

If that isn't possible then get it home and take it straight up to your bedroom – without removing the plastic packaging.

Try it out for at least ten minutes in your normal sleep position. Not for comfort. Of course it's going to feel plastic and strange. But check whether you can feel your neck tipping forward or backwards.

If you do, or if you feel any other niggle or pain, then whip straight back to the store brandishing your pillow and receipt and get a refund or an exchange.

Another thing to consider (and this is about helping you avoid another sort of pain) is what sort of care your pillow will need.

Some are OK to put through the washing machine. Others are dry clean only. Some can only be put through particular types of washing machine.

Read the label before you buy, because it will last longer if you care for it properly. But be realistic about how much caring for it you will actually do.

Finally on pillow selection, don't make an assumption that the type of pillow you have used up until now will still suit you.

Our bodies change as they age. We put on weight. We lose weight. We pick up new aches and pains. Check each and every time that the pillow type you are buying is still right for you now.

Good luck with finding the right pillow for you! It's out there somewhere...

Now, onto the best sleep position for your aching neck.

As ever, the best position you can sleep in is on your back. If you can do this it might be worth adding a small neck roll into the pillow case of a softer pillow so both your head and your neck are individually supported.

Try to ensure that the curve of your neck when you are lying down is similar to that when you are standing with a good posture.

Side sleeping is the next best option. As we've already mentioned, make sure that your pillow is no thicker than six inches.

But bear in mind that your height and the width of your shoulders will have an impact on what is right for you.

For example, if you are very petite you will need a slimmer pillow than if you have very broad shoulders.

As a rule of thumb (or perhaps neck...) the height of your pillow should match the width of one shoulder to keep you happily in alignment.

Finally – stomach sleeping. You know what I'm going to say by now. This position will place more strain on your neck than any other.

Try to break the habit (I know how hard this will be) or go without a pillow altogether.

There is one thing that most of us do in bed that will be causing trouble for your neck.

And that is (perhaps more innocently than you had been thinking) looking at your phone.

Most of us will spend at least a few minutes scrolling through messages or checking Facebook or Twitter – or just surfing the net.

But here is the mathematics of what that is doing to your neck…

Your neck muscles are designed to support your head in a neutral position. When in a good posture your neck is dealing with around 10-12 pounds of force.

But the moment you look down at your phone your head can plunge by around sixty degrees. And that throws sixty pounds of force onto your muscles, tendons and ligaments.

So try to ditch your phone in bed or, if you have to check, hold it directly up in front of your eyes.

It is worth mentioning that the blue-ish light that the screen emits is scientifically proven to inhibit the amount of sleep hormone, melatonin.

I know that little fact isn't directly connected with solving your aches and pains – but it should help you get a better night's sleep. So I thought I'd throw it in.

Other things that can help you get the sleep you deserve are to consider using one of those u-shaped travel pillows.

Primarily designed to help people snatch forty winks on a plane they can also have benefit when you are sitting up, reading or watching television.

They offer more support to your neck muscles… although beware of those that bulge too much at the back and push your head forward.

Applied heat for ten to fifteen minutes can also make it easier to slip into bed without pain. Consider having a shower or a bath and letting your cares (and pain) slide away.

It is worth relaxing and stretching your neck to loosen the muscles before you get into bed to sleep.

Be careful how you do these because you clearly don't want to do anything that makes your pain worse or ends up placing extra stress on your body.

Here is one that you can try to stretch out the tenseness of the day...

Stand next to a wall with around twelve inches between it and your shoulders.

Raise your arms high above your head, stretching out as far as you can go.

Angle your arms towards the wall so your elbow and the palm of your hand are flat against it.

Then turn your head away from the wall, bringing your chin down towards the floor until you feel a slight stretch in the back of your neck.

Put your other hand on top of your head, pulling it forward to emphasise the stretch.

Hold it for between thirty and sixty seconds.

But, of course, stop if you feel pain at any point.

Try treating your neck pain with anti-inflammatories in the first instance too. They may give you the help you need to drift off.

Any neck pain that lasts for more than a week needs to be referred to a doctor.

Partly this is to check that there is nothing else going on that needs to be properly diagnosed. But mostly this is to ensure that you are getting the best treatment regime you possibly can.

They may well be able to refer you to a physiotherapist or other physical trainer who will be able to teach you more stretches or exercises to get your neck back into alignment.

Whatever happens next... good luck! And have a good night's sleep!

HAS THIS BOOK HELPED YOU?

If this book has helped you then please consider leaving a review on Amazon.

It means other people are more likely to find it and read about the ways that they can help reduce their back pain.

Thank you!

www.ingramcontent.com/pod-product-compliance
Lightning Source LLC
Chambersburg PA
CBHW061928270726
48660CB00003BA/1097